MW00899159

It Shouldn't Hurt

to

Nurse Your Baby

Breastfeeding Solutions for the
Six Most Common Causes of Painful Nipples

Lisa Paladino CNM, IBCLC

It Shouldn't Hurt to Nurse Your Baby

Breastfeeding Solutions for the Six Most Common Causes of Painful Nipples

Lisa Paladino CNM, IBLC

Photo credit: Cover Kelley McCarthy Downer

Editor: Michele Nichols MS

Graphic Design: Russ Paladino

ISBN-10: 1545410259

ISBN-13: 978-1545410257

This book is offered for educational and informational purposes only and should not be used as a replacement for the medical advice of your health care provider. All efforts have been made to ensure the accuracy of the information as of the date published. The author and publisher disclaim responsibility for any adverse effects arising from the use or application of the information contained herein.

DEDICATION

I dedicate this book to all of the women that I have met who have shared their breastfeeding journey with me. It is an honor to be with families at this most vulnerable, yet transformative time in life. I can only hope that they have learned half as much from me as I have learned from them.

What I have learned is this: women are strong! I have witnessed women become mothers and blossom in amazing ways. The power of breastfeeding is something that few expect, but many experience.

My wish for you, as you read this book, is to realize that any bumps and roadblocks that you face are worth the effort. The beginning sometimes feels like forever, but it's only the start. Take one feeding, one day at a time. The rewards for getting through the tough times are worth it. Breastmilk is magical and nursing your baby is an experience that you both deserve to enjoy.

Cherish every moment!

It Shouldn't Hurt to Nurse Your Baby

TABLE OF CONTENTS

It Shouldn't Hurt to Nurse Your Baby

A note about gender:

In this book the baby will be referred to as she for no other reason than convenience- no offense to the boys.

It Shouldn't Hurt to Nurse Your Baby

INTRODUCTION:

Congratulations!

Breastfeeding can be one of the most rewarding and empowering experiences of your lifetime. You have gotten through pregnancy and birth- you thought that would be the hard part. You have read about breastfeeding, maybe took a class, maybe joined a support group online. You have decided to nourish your child as she is meant to be fed- at your breast. You thought you were prepared with all that you needed to know. And then, for some of us, when baby feeds - it hurts! How or why can this natural process be so painful?

Well, actually, it shouldn't hurt. There are many old wive's tails surrounding breastfeeding, and one of these is that it "always hurts in the beginning". Moms come into my practice saying that it hurts, but not too much and "it's supposed to, right?". To be honest, this makes me angry. Why would a physiologic process that we have to do to survive hurt our mothers? I doubt there is any natural process that men do that we'd say the same thing about. Some minor discomfort? Maybe. Pain, cracking, bleeding? Not normal. Ok, rant over. Bottom line is that pain is an indicator that something isn't quite right and there are steps to take to make it more comfortable and easier for your baby. An important fact to remember is that comfort while feeding is not just for you. If latch hurts, chances are that your baby isn't nursing effectively and she will not get as much milk as she should.

Nipple soreness can start at birth, can slowly get worse over time, or can start at any point during the nursing relationship. My goal is for you to understand why it hurts and what you can do to change the cause, heal your nipples and go on to reach your breastfeeding goals.

This book is based on my personal experience helping women to nurse for years, first as a RN in the hospital- working on the mother/baby and labor and delivery units, then as a midwife, and now in my private practice as a lactation consultant. I continue to learn and evolve my recommendations based on new information.

What I have included in these pages is what I currently suggest to the women who come to my practice who are experiencing pain. Some of what I have learned is from tradition, some from formal education, some from other lactation professionals and health care providers, and some from women who have shared what has worked for them. I have not included commercial products, as in most cases, I do not find them necessary. I am a minimalist. I find that the less we interfere with the natural process of feeding, the easier it is. Actually, I sometimes find that using "nipple products" prevents healing. This doesn't mean that I don't think that using a commercial product is ever necessary. It is only that I don't use them as first line of treatment. I don't recommend that moms use them instead of seeking professional guidance.

It is possible to nurse comfortably and enjoy the experience! In this book you will learn the most common reasons that breast-feeding might hurt and the actions to take when it does. I have not listed all of the reasons why breastfeeding can cause pain, or exclaim that I have all of the solutions. This is not the only book on breastfeeding that you will need, as there is so much more to learn on the subject. The six causes of nipple pain correlate with the chapter numbers. They are: latch, tethered oral tissues, engorgement, nipple infection, nipple bleb/milk blister, and vasospasm.

What this book is not- it is not a replacement for "in person" lactation support or medical care. Nipple pain may be a sign that baby isn't eating enough at the breast or that you have an infection requiring medical treatment. Either case is not to be ignored.

If you have any concerns that are not quickly solved by the suggestions in this book, call your health care provider and find a local IBCLC (International Board Certified Lactation Consultant) for an evaluation. You may need both a medical professional and a lactation specialist. They are not always one in the same. Do not assume that your health care provider understands how to help you with breastfeeding problems. While your provider may support breastfeeding on a philosophical level, she may lack the knowledge to guide you through challenges. This is through no fault of the provider. Unfortunately, lactation is not a topic that is taught comprehensively in most medical school, residency curriculums, nursing or midwifery programs. A sad example of this is that when I took my midwifery boards I actually had to chose an answer on the test that I knew was wrong, but it was what my texts and test prep had taught me. Frustrating paradox, but truth!

I often get the question- "An IBCL-what?". At the time of the writing of this book, I only know of a handful of other IBCLCs in the borough of NY that I live in. It's a profession that is in its early stages, so I'm not shocked that most people have never heard of, or met someone, who does what I do.

So what exactly is an International Board Certified Lactation Consultant?

An IBCLC is a healthcare professional who has completed extensive education in health sciences and human lactation and has unique and documented experience working with nursing mothers. She specializes in the clinical management of breastfeeding and is trained to recognize when it is appropriate to refer to a doctor for further treatment. She must abide by Professional Standards and re-certify every five years. There are many types of "lactation consultants". Please be aware that an IBCLC is the highest certification level to be achieved in breastfeeding. While other designations may have their role, an IBCLC is the provider of choice when simple breastfeeding solutions do not provide relief.

When seeking a lactation professional, be sure to ask the type of training and certification of the consultant. Under the Affordable Care Act, all women in the United States are entitled to a consultation by an IBCLC, covered by medical insurance.

Important Information, no matter the cause of the pain:

ALWAYS FEED THE BABY

If your nipples hurt so much that you cannot nurse the baby, feed the baby in an alternate manner. First choice is with your expressed breastmilk, but if that is not possible, feed with donor breastmilk, or a breastmilk substitute (formula) as recommended by your pediatrician. The first rule of breastfeeding is "Feed the baby". It is risky to not feed the baby in order to exclusively breastfeed when the baby cannot feed at the breast. Baby may be fed by bottle, cup, spoon, syringe or supplemental nursing system. Lactation Consultants can guide you on what options are best for your specific situation.

Please note:

If your baby is supplemented, pumping is important in order to build and preserve your milk supply. It will also prevent discomfort and clogged ducts which can lead to infection. It is recommended to pump every time your baby takes a feeding other than at your breast. This includes all bottle, cup, or syringe feedings.

A word about pumping and nipple pain:

Pumping shouldn't hurt your nipples. I refer to nursing in this book, because most cases of nipple pain are caused by at the breast feeding. However, I don't mean to ignore the moms who pump exclusively, regularly or occasionally. Most of the information in this book will apply for nipple pain while pumping as well, but the solution is often easier. If pumping hurts or causes nipple trauma, try different size flanges (the horn-like part that goes onto your nipple). If the fit isn't right, it can cause pain and nipple breakdown. Using lubrication, such as coconut oil in the flanges often helps. If it continues to hurt, please reach out to an IBCLC.

Comfort measures for nipples:

✦ Letting expressed breastmilk remain on your nipple after feedings can help them heal since your breastmilk has antibacterial and antifungal properties.

✦ When possible, leave your bra off or the flaps open to allow air flow to your nipples. If you are using breast pads, be sure to change them frequently. Washable cotton is preferred over disposable pads.

✦ Organic, food-grade coconut or olive oil can be safely used on your nipples to soothe them and prevent infection. Of course, do not use these oils if you know that you have an allergy to them.

✦ Nipples can be washed gently with mild soapy water before nursing using non-perfumed, non-antibacterial soap and rinsing well before feeding.

✦ Saline soaks also help healing: dissolve 1 teaspoon of salt in 8 ounces of warm water and use a clean washcloth or gauze pad to place the saline solution onto your nipples.

When to call your healthcare provider:

✦ If baby is not feeding between 8-12 times in each 24 hour period or is feeding constantly without ever seeming to be be satisfied.

✦ If baby is not having wet diapers as expected at her age: 1 on day 1, 2 on day 2, 3 on day 3, 4 on day 4, 5 on day 5, and 6 or more on all days after that.

✦ Baby is not having dirty diapers as expected at her age:1 on day 1, 2 on day 2, 3 or more from day 3 on. Stool starts out black and sticky, will get lighter, from brown to greenish to yellow and seedy by day 5. It is never "normal" for a baby to miss bowel movements.

✦ Baby's skin or eyes appear yellow (jaundice).

✦ Baby is very sleepy and never wakes up on her own to feed

✦ Your nipples are cracked and bleeding or have any pus or discharge.

✦ You have any redness, warmth, or pain in your breasts accompanied by fever over 101°F and flu-like symptoms such as headache, muscle aches, and fatigue.

✦ You have any doubt that something isn't right. Trust your instinct and call for help, even if it's just for reassurance.

CHAPTER 1:

LATCH

As a lactation consultant, I find that the most common cause for nipple pain while breastfeeding is a poor latch. The good news is, that this may be simple to fix.

Latch refers to how your baby attaches to your breast to feed. If she is not positioned correctly for latch, it can cause discomfort and nipple trauma. Compression can be caused by holding the baby in a way that doesn't allow your nipple to reach the soft palate in the back of your baby's mouth. When the nipple is at the correct angle, and deep enough to reach the soft palate, it is usually comfortable and it allows her to transfer milk efficiently.

The goal of the latch is to have your nipple land as far back as possible in your baby's mouth, but how do you achieve that? The key is to have the baby latch to you, instead of you trying to latch her onto your nipple/breast. It may seem as though that is the same, but it is not. Most babies know how to latch instinctually. The less we do to get in the way, the easier it is for them.

You may notice that there is no mention of using a 'boppy" or other such nursing pillow. I personally feel that these pillows interfere with an baby being able to obtain a good latch. If you would like to use a pillow, use it to support your arms or baby's back after she is latched to the breast, but not while you are positioning her.

Skin to skin

In order to achieve a comfortable, safe and effective latch try skin to skin. Skin to skin means having only a diaper on baby and that you are disrobed from the waist up. If you are worried about keeping baby warm, a light blanket over her will be fine. Skin to skin is always the best way to feed baby, especially while you are both learning how to feed. It allows her to hear your heart beating and your voice through your chest as she recently heard when she was in your womb. The reason that skin to skin assists latch is that it allows your baby to use the primitive reflexes that she is born with to find your breast and attach correctly. Babies up to 12 weeks of age have the instinct to find the nipple and self-attach if left alone. It is so amazing to realize that your baby knows exactly what to do! Skin to skin also helps to regulate her blood sugar, temperature, and mood. Putting her skin to skin on your chest can calm her down if she is frustrated or crying at the breast and having trouble settling down. It will also calm you to have her there. Take some deep breaths and enjoy holding your baby close to you.

While skin to skin, laying back in a semi-reclining position, with your baby placed high on your chest and letting her find your nipple can make things easiest. Whatever position is comfortable for you can work for skin to skin.

Laid back breastfeeding

If you are laying back, baby may bop up and down in a searching type motion. Try not to interfere, but support her back as she moves so that she is safe. Some babies move rather quickly and are stronger than you might expect! Resist the urge to help out, she knows where she's going. She may stop along the way, but as long as she's not crying, let her move down to the nipple on her own. It is so amazing to watch this happen!

Sitting or Side Lying

If you are sitting up, or lying on your side, make sure that you are in a comfortable position. Bring the baby to you, not you to baby so that you are not leaning over her. You will be in this position for a bit of time, so you want to be careful that your back and neck aren't strained.

Some guiding principles that work in all positions:

✦ Nothing should come between you and baby; no blankets or thick clothing. Sometimes bras can get in the way. Be sure that nothing is preventing baby from getting close to you.

✦ Do not try to feed her while she is swaddled. She needs to have her hands free to hug your breast in order to get close enough. One hand should be on either side of your breast. Babies often use their hands to help with nursing and get frustrated when swaddled.

✦ Hold your baby close and securely, but not too tightly. Do not hold her head, instead support her neck so that she can tilt her head back to come onto the breast. Try not to touch her head at all while she is latching.

✦ When you look down at her, she should be belly to belly with you. Let her completely face you, with her head, neck shoulders, belly, hips and legs lined up, not twisted.

✦ When you are holding your baby in a comfortable position, tickle the space between her upper lip and her nose with your nipple, do not push your nipple into baby's mouth or baby's mouth onto the nipple. Allow her to move her head back and open her mouth wide. When she opens wide, hug her close to you with a gentle hold on her upper back.

✦ Be sure that your baby's feet are supported, either by your hands, a pillow, rolled up blanket or the back of the seat you are on. Many babies won't nurse if they don't feel secure. Sometimes touching the bottom of the feet is what gets the baby to open wide to latch.

✦ Remember, whatever position you choose, never hold or touch the baby's head with your hands or arms while she is trying to latch. Support low on her neck and upper back instead so that she can move her head freely to latch on. Babies latch best when they can come up to the nipple to latch by tilting the head back. I know that I am repeating myself, but I often find that moms want to hold the baby's head and this can really cause difficulty for some babies (and their mom's nipples). When you touch a baby's head she automatically tucks her chin in towards her chest, and for an ideal latch, her chin needs to be up and against your breast.

✦ When baby is latched and positioned correctly, her chin should be against your breast with her head slightly tipped back so that her nose is not "squished" into the breast.

✦ Once baby is latched, be sure that her lips are flanged out (not sucked in) on the top and bottom. If not, try to help her by flipping them out with your finger. You may want to gently tug down on baby's chin. This can help baby to open a bit wider on the breast which will bring more comfort.

✦ If the latch hurts for more than a few seconds (count to 10), unlatch her and start over. The safest way to do that is to put your finger in baby's mouth to break the seal and then gently remove your nipple.

If you can't find a comfortable hold or position that allows your baby to nurse without causing you pain, please reach out to an IBCLC (International Board Certified Lactation Consultant) for an evaluation.

CHAPTER 2:

TETHERED ORAL TISSUES: LIP, TONGUE AND BUCCAL TIES

Tethered Oral Tissues are abnormally formed or tight attachments in the mouth that prevent functional movement. There are three types that seem to effect breastfeeding: Lip (maxillary), tongue (linguinal) and cheek (buccal). The band of tissue that attaches the tongue to the bottom of the mouth and the lip to the gum line, is called a frenum or frenulum. The lip frenum can be too far down on the gum line or too thick or tight to allow the lip to curl outward. The frenum under the tongue can be either too short, thick, or tight or it can be attached in a position that holds the tongue too close to the floor of the mouth. Frenums found in the cheek area can cause pulling from the gum to the inside of the mouth, preventing the baby from opening to a wide gape.

In order to feed comfortably and effectively, a baby needs to be able to open her mouth to a wide gape, lift her tongue and move it in a way that draws the nipple in and creates an effective pull of milk from the nipple. If there is a lip, tongue or buccal tie, it may interfere with the ability to do this efficiently.

Often, tethered oral tissues will be the cause of the latching difficulties addressed in the previous chapter. If you have tried all of the suggestions to improve latch in Chapter 1, and feeding is still hurting your nipples, consider that there may be a tie preventing a comfortable latch.

Tongue, lip, and buccal ties can prevent the baby from coordinating the suck and swallow that is needed to transfer milk from your breast. The baby who has a restriction like this may appear to be sucking constantly, but only stops to swallow occasionally. These are babies who need to feed constantly, without ever seeming to be satisfied. They may have slow weight gain.

Other babies with oral restrictions may have difficulty handling flow of milk and bite/pull back on the nipple or choke when mom has a let-down of milk. And still others are gaining well, or even seeming to gain really quickly, but they have upset tummies. These babies have moms that have compensated with an overabundant milk supply. They don't have to work very hard to get the "easy" milk from mom and they gulp it down very fast, then get frustrated after the initial let-down and the milk flow slows.

Besides causing pain for you, there may be other symptoms that you notice in your baby. When a baby can't move her tongue well, or open her mouth fully for a latch, she will swallow more air than she should. This air can result in gas pains (colic), spitting up (reflux), and explosive stools. While these symptoms do not occur in all babies with oral restrictions, they are possibilities to be aware of.

Tethered oral tissues may also have implications for later in life. The position of the tongue in the mouth is responsible for the formation of the palate, the shape of the skull and the airway, so this is not just a concern for breastfeeding.

Some babies breastfeed without a problem, but go on to have difficulty drinking from a bottle or cup. They may have trouble chewing and swallowing solid foods, develop orthodontic issues, speech problems or airway issues (such as snoring and sleep apnea).

If any of these scenarios seem familiar to you, please have your baby evaluated for tethered oral tissues. A word of caution about diagnosis of tethered oral tissues: This is not the type of diagnosis that should be made from a picture on social media. There are many groups on Facebook that are dedicated to the subject. Some babies may appear to have a tie, but they have normal function of their tongues and mouths. This is a diagnosis of form and function Tongue, lip and buccal ties are best identified by an IBCLC or any other health care provider that has pursued education and training to recognize such issues and can guide you on the best way to achieve release of the oral tightness.

Many pediatricians may miss this during exam because their education may not have included how oral structures effect breastfeeding. This is especially true in locations where there have been a few generations of babies who have been fed by bottle. As a Registered Nurse, a Certified Nurse Midwife or as an IBCLC, this was not a part of my education. Those of us proficient in this diagnosis know what we do about it because we have had pursued continuing education about it.

Treatment of the ties may include revision (cutting or laser treatment of the frenum), body work, and oral exercises. My preference is an evaluation by a specialist who can release the frenum using a laser in an office setting.

The office procedure for release of ties is most successful when thought of as part of a plan set out by your IBCLC who understands how the tongue functions in breastfeeding and what other treatment modalities should be recommended. She knows how to help your baby learn to latch effectively after revision. She can provide anticipatory guidance and recommendations regarding analgesia. She will also guide you to the best methods for adjusting other concerns that may have developed due to the latch, such as milk supply and nipple pain issues.

CHAPTER 3:

ENGORGEMENT

Normal engorgement is the fullness that you feel when your milk is changing from the initial milk (called colostrum) to mature milk. The change usually occurs between days three and five after birth, but can occur later if baby isn't nursing well or if you have had a premature birth, a difficult labor with lots of interventions or a cesarean section. Engorgement isn't always noticeable. Sometimes it is minor and doesn't cause any issues, but often it can make your breasts and nipples sore. Some women describe it as fullness or tightness, but sometimes the breasts may feel very hard, hot to the touch, and painful. It may be accompanied by a low grade fever, which isn't by itself a sign of infection, but should be watched closely.

During these first few days and weeks, your milk supply is regulating- your body is learning to make exactly the amount of milk that your baby will need for the first few months and beyond. For this reason and to prevent engorgement from lasting beyond a day or two, it is important not to pump unless there is a medical indication or a reason that baby can't be fed directly. It is also not recommended to give your baby an artificial nipple (bottle or pacifier) during the first 3-4 weeks while your body is setting the amount of milk your baby needs.

Another cause for engorgement that can occur at any time during your breastfeeding journey is missing a feeding. This can happen when your baby first starts sleeping through the night, or if you have to be away from the baby and you don't remember to express your milk.

It is important to realize that there is a difference between engorgement and mastitis. Engorgement is a normal and expected physiologic change. It occurs in both breasts, and is not accompanied by any other symptoms. Mastitis is an infection of the breast. It is usually in one breast, not both. It is painful to touch, and the area of the breast that is affected is red and hot to touch. The milk output from that breast may be decreased. Mastitis is accompanied by fever over 101°F, and flu-like symptoms, such as fatigue, body aches and headache. If you have any of the signs of mastitis, please call your healthcare provider because you may need to be treated with antibiotics to clear the infection.

The reason that I include engorgement as a cause for nipple pain can is that the nipple may be stretched out and flattened by the fullness of the breast. Not only is this painful, but it may make it hard for your baby to get a good latch. She may cause discomfort as she attempts to get her mouth around a nipple that isn't protruding as it once did.

If your breasts are so full that baby cannot latch on, try to hand express a small amount of milk in order to release the fullness that is flattening your nipples. You can also use your finger tips to firmly press around the areola (dark area surrounding your nipples) to allow your nipples to "come out" before you allow the baby to latch.

The best way to prevent and treat engorgement is to feed your baby on demand, at least 8-12 times in 24 hours. Allow the baby to nurse on one side for as long as she wants, then offer the other side. If she doesn't nurse on both sides during a feeding and you still feel uncomfortably full, you can hand express to comfort or use a breast soak. The reason that you don't want to pump to relieve engorgement (if the baby is able to nurse) is because the pump will cause more stimulation and then the discomfort of engorgement will continue for a longer period of time.

Breast soak:

To soak your breasts to relieve engorgement, fill a basin with the warmest water you can stand to touch and lean over it, putting your breasts into the water. Use gravity and have your breasts completely covered in the warm water. While your breasts are soaking, gently massage your breasts from your armpits towards your nipple and in the opposite direction. This should express milk into the water and help you to feel relieved without stimulation that can lead to increased milk production.

For comfort before a feed, warm soaks help, but after a feeding, cold may feel better. This can be in the form of a cold washcloth, an ice pack, or cold cabbage leaves.

As a reminder: if you have fever over 101°F, flu-like symptoms, redness, or warmth concentrated on one area of the breast or if you cannot feed the baby, contact your health care provider and IBCLC for further assistance.

CHAPTER 4:

NIPPLE INFECTION: BACTERIAL & YEAST

There are two different types of nipple infection that can happen when a mom is breastfeeding. Nipples can be infected by either bacteria or yeast (also known as candida). Both are very painful and require treatment.

There are differences between the two types of infections. Bacterial infections usually start with, and are accompanied by, cracked nipples. This type of infection is often associated with early breastfeeding. Treatment of baby is not usually required and the appropriate treatment for mom usually resolves the condition within a few days.

Nipples that are infected by yeast don't always appear to be cracked. It is not typical for a yeast infection to occur in the first few weeks. This type of infection usually occurs with established breastfeeding. If there is a maternal yeast infection, treatment of the baby is almost always required. Also, it is important that all pump supplies, and anything baby may have used in her mouth, such as nipples or pacifiers, be cleaned properly to prevent cross contamination and reinfection.
Yeast can become chronic, and it can take a very long time to rid both mom and baby of symptoms.

Bacterial Nipple Infection:

If you are a new mom with cracked, bleeding nipples, accompanied by redness around the nipple, yellow crust or pussy drainage, it is likely that you have a bacterial infection. When poor latch leads to cracked nipples, it is very easy to get an infection of the nipple due to overgrowth of bacteria that normally live on our skin.

Cracked nipples may heal with at-home interventions and improving latch, but if you have any concern that your cracked nipples are infected, please call your healthcare provider/IBCLC. Your provider may want to treat with a topical antibiotic ointment. The most serious concern of untreated bacterial infection of the nipple is that the bacteria can pass through the nipple into the breast and cause mastitis (breast infection).

Symptoms of mastitis include a painful, hot, red area on the breast and fever or flu-like symptoms. These symptoms require medical evaluation.

Comfort measures for nipples:

✦ Letting expressed breastmilk remain on your nipple after feedings can help them heal since your breastmilk has antibacterial and antifungal properties.

✦ When possible, leave your bra off or the flaps open to allow air flow to your nipples. If you are using breast pads, be sure to change them frequently

✦ Organic, food-grade coconut or olive oil can be safely used on your nipples to soothe them and prevent infection. Of course, do not use these oils if you know that you have an allergy to them.

✦ Nipples can be washed gently with mild soapy water before nursing using non-perfumed, non-antibacterial soap and rinsing well before feeding.

✦ Saline soaks also help healing: dissolve 1 teaspoon of salt in 8 ounces of warm water and use a clean washcloth or gauze pad to place the saline solution onto your nipples.

If you have cracked or bleeding nipples, with or without infection, treating the nipples is vital, but improving your latch to prevent further damage to your nipples is also important. Finding the cause of the pain and reversing it will prevent further damage and allow your nipples to heal.

Yeast (Candida) Infections:

Yeast (candida) is normally present on our skin, but situations that cause an imbalance in the microbiome can cause the yeast to overgrow and cause symptoms. This can happen after use of antibiotic by mom or baby or during times of stress and high sugar intake.

Nipples infected by yeast (candida) tend to be red, shiny, itchy, or scaly (but this varies) and very painful to touch. Nursing may range from being mildly uncomfortable to being excruciatingly painful. Candida infection is sometimes accompanied by burning or shooting pain in the breast that can radiate to the armpit or back. Often, but not always, there may be a white patches on baby's tongue or in her mouth. Baby may also have diaper rash. Sometimes baby shows no sign of infection.

The topical comfort measures listed above (under bacterial infection) may provide relief, specifically the use of coconut oil. Coconut oil has antifungal properties and may be tried for a few days for mild cases. A rinse with a solution of one cup of water plus one tablespoon of apple cider vinegar and then air drying nipples may help to fight the candida. However, in many cases, a yeast infection requires medical evaluation of mom and baby. There are anti-yeast medications that may be prescribed to be used topically and sometimes internally. Nutritional support, especially removing sugar and yeast from the diet, and adding a probiotic, may help bring the microbiome back into balance and stop the flare of candida.

CHAPTER 5:

NIPPLE BLEBS/MILK BLISTERS

If you are experiencing pain on one nipple, and you see an enlarged pore or white spot, it may be a milk blister. This is also known as a nipple bleb ("bleb"). The pain may range from mildly uncomfortable to excruciating and even prevent you from allowing your baby to nurse. The bleb may appear to get smaller and larger, go away and return.

Blebs are clogged ducts that appear on the nipple. If you think of the milk duct as a tube, like a straw, the bleb is a clog at the opening of the straw. When the milk sits in the "tube" for a period of time, and it isn't cleared, a layer of the skin of your nipple may grow over the blocked milk. The pain that you feel is the pressure of the milk trying to come out and not being able to because the passage is blocked. If you understand it in this way, the treatment will make sense. You must get rid of the clog to get the milk flowing again. It is vital to remove milk by nursing, hand expressing or pumping, because the pain will only increase if the clog isn't cleared. Also, if a blocked duct remains, milk will collect in the milk duct which can lead to swelling of that duct, and possible mastitis (breast infection). Treatment that you can try at home includes methods that will soften the skin of the bleb and remove it in order to get the milk flowing again. It is advisable to wash your hands before touching the nipple when you have a bleb.

For pain relief of pain caused by a bleb:

✦ Saline soak: 1 tsp of salt (Epsom salt or sea salt) in 8 ounces of warm water applied to your nipple with a gauze pad or clean washcloth. The warmest water you can touch will feel best, but be careful not to burn yourself, nipples have sensitive skin. This is especially helpful before nursing.

✦ Application of olive oil or coconut oil to the nipple with careful massage of the area of the bleb. If you can, rub gently at the borders of the bleb to try to remove the skin that is covering it.

✦ If these methods do not provide relief, or if you have any sign of nipple or breast infection, see your health care provider as soon as possible. In some cases, a needle may need to be used to open the bleb, but that should only be done by a health care provider under sterile conditions as it can easily lead to infection. If you have the bleb opened by needle, the soaks and oil may be helpful to keep it from happening again.

✦ If you experience frequent milk blebs or one that keeps getting blocked, there is a supplement called sunflower lecithin that may be helpful to prevent the formation of clogs in the milk ducts. You can discuss this with your health care provider.

CHAPTER 6:

NIPPLE VASOSPASM

Some women experience blanching of the nipple after nursing, usually immediately after baby comes off of the nipple. It is described as intense burning pain, and the nipple may appear to turn deep purple or white.

As in all forms of pain, it is important not only to treat the symptoms, but to find the cause in order to stop the pain from occurring. This type of pain may be the result of a poor latch or oral restrictions. Because of this, it is recommended that you adjust the latch and/or get a professional evaluation of your baby's oral anatomy in order to prevent further nipple trauma.

Treatments for immediate relief of blanching nipples:

✦ Covering the nipple immediately after taking the baby off, in order to prevent exposure to cold air.

✦ Using a warmed, food grade oil (coconut and olive work well) on the nipple after feeding.

✦ Applying a warm, wet compress to the nipple immediately after feeding.

A more severe form of blanching of the nipple can be caused by the vasospasm of Raynaud's disease. Raynaud's isn't specifically a breastfeeding syndrome, but it can effect multiple areas of the body. Those with Raynaud's typically have fingers and toes that react to cold and stress with a feeling of numbness and reduced blood flow. Women who are prone to Raynaud's phenomena may have this effect their nipples as well. The treatments mentioned above, for blanching nipples, usually help relieve Raynaud's vasospasm as well, although in extreme cases, a medication may be needed.

As in all lactation difficulties, your first call should be to an IBCLC (International Board Certified Lactation Consultant) to find if simple adjustments to latch and position can relieve your symptoms. If not, please reach out for medical assistance.

IN CONCLUSION

I sincerely hope that the information on the preceding pages will assist you to meet your personal breastfeeding goals. Your success is my inspiration!

If you are in need of further information, have questions or hints to add or would like to join my community, please reach out.

Contact information:

Website:

www.StatenIslandBreastfeeding.com or

www.LisaMariePaladino.com

Email: Lisa@StatenIslandBreastfeeding.com

Facebook:

https://www.facebook.com/LisaPaladinoMidwifeLactation/

https://www.facebook.com/groups/RootsSI/

With Much Love,

Lisa

WITH GRATITUDE...

I would like to thank my children (Andrew, Jessica and Jillian) and Godchildren (Samantha, Victoria, Alex and Kayla). Each of them, in their individual ways, taught me how to mother and how to nurse (or not). The experiences of their births, their first years and our feeding relationships forever influence my counseling of new moms. Special thanks to my husband, Russ, without whose support, nothing I do would be possible. I am who I am because of him.

Only the family of another lactation consultant or midwife would understand the conversations, textbooks, flyers and models that are ever present due to my work. I appreciate the patience of my entire family to put up with sometimes embarrassing situations.

To my IBCLC "sisters" Rebeca Four IBCLC and Michelle Farfel IBCLC- thanks for always being a just a message away with your wisdom, experience and humor. Being able to learn from you both has made my mission easier.

To Dr. Scott Siegel, Dr. Jennifer Falcone, and Dr. Jackie Hines- I am so grateful for our professional collaboration and for your friendship. I think we make a great team!

To my "breast" friend, Joan Greenberg RN, IBCLC without whom I wouldn't be a lactation consultant. I never take your love and support for granted. We have learned so much together!

To my mentor, Marianne DiStefano RN, IBCLC. You helped form my professional identity. You believed in my dreams before I understood them. I treasure the role you played in my life and the memories of the work we did together.

Joni and Marianne, our journey didn't go as planned, but we got as far as circumstances would allow. I continue *our* mission, in a different direction but with the same motivation, one mother/baby dyad at a time.

ABOUT THE AUTHOR

Professional: Lisa Paladino is an International Board Certified Lactation Consultant/Certified Nurse Midwife in Staten Island, NY. Lisa's 30 year career includes 28 years of hospital experience, first as an RN, then as a CNM, and finally as an IBCLC. In 2015 Lisa founded **Staten Island Lactation and Wellness** to provide private practice care for women's lactation, nutrition and wellness needs with an approach that integrates the Midwifery and functional medicine models. Her mission is to empower women to reach their health goals through guidance, education and community. Lisa trusts the innate wisdom of women to know what feels right for themselves and for their children. Her goal is to change the culture around baby feeding and wellness, one mother/baby dyad at a time. Lisa enjoys engaging in social media forums and public speaking to share her message and assist women to rise to reclaim the benefits of a healthy lifestyle in a world that makes it challenging to do so.

Personal: Lisa has been married for 30 wonderful years to her husband and soul mate, Russ, and has three beautiful children and four wonderful Godchildren that continuously amaze her with their talents and individuality. Lisa's motivation to change the culture of baby feeding comes from her own experience as a new mom. She remembers feeling like something wasn't right when her newborn babies were taken from the room soon after birth, and being devastated when told that she didn't have enough milk by a pediatrician who didn't understand the biological imperative of breastfeeding. When pregnant the third time, Lisa started learning all about how breastfeeding should work and decided that nothing would stop her. That home-birthed baby (who was born with a cleft lip) nursed exclusively from birth and weaned when she decided to.

Made in the USA
Columbia, SC
14 May 2017